DR. BARBARA 7-DAY FULL-BODY DETOX

Transform your health: Dr. Barbara's 7-days full-body detox, rejuvenate, cleanse and energize with nature's healing power

I0781582

Miguel Sofia

Table of Contents

COPYRIGHT © 2023

CHAPTER ONE

Introduction to Dr. Barbara's Herbal Full-Body Detox Program

Dr. Barbara's Herbal Full-Body Detox Program is a comprehensive and holistic approach to cleansing and rejuvenating the body using natural herbs and botanicals. Developed by Dr. Barbara, a renowned herbalist and naturopathic doctor, this program aims to support the body's natural detoxification processes, promote overall health and well-being, and restore balance to the body.

Detoxification has become increasingly popular in recent years as people seek ways to rid their bodies of accumulated toxins and pollutants from the environment, diet, and lifestyle factors. Dr. Barbara's Herbal Full-Body Detox Program offers a safe and effective way to cleanse the body without resorting to extreme measures or harsh chemicals.

This program is based on the principles of traditional herbal medicine, which has been used for centuries to support detoxification and promote health. By harnessing the power of medicinal plants and herbs, Dr. Barbara's program provides a gentle yet effective way to eliminate toxins, support organ function, and enhance overall vitality.

In this detailed exploration, we will delve into the key components of Dr. Barbara's Herbal Full-Body Detox Program, including its philosophy, methodology, and the specific herbs and botanicals used. We will also discuss the potential benefits of detoxification, how the program works, and important considerations to keep in mind before embarking on a detox journey.

Philosophy of Dr. Barbara's Herbal Full-Body Detox Program

At the heart of Dr. Barbara's Herbal Full-Body Detox Program is the belief that the body has an innate ability to heal and rejuvenate itself when given the right support and resources. Rather than focusing solely on symptom management, this program takes a holistic approach to health and wellness, addressing the root causes of imbalance and toxicity.

The philosophy of this detox program is rooted in the principles of naturopathic medicine, which emphasizes the importance of supporting the body's natural healing mechanisms and addressing the underlying imbalances that contribute to disease and dysfunction. By providing the body with the necessary nutrients, herbs, and botanicals, Dr. Barbara's program aims to enhance detoxification pathways, support organ function, and promote overall vitality.

Central to the philosophy of Dr. Barbara's program is the idea that detoxification is not a one-time event but rather an ongoing process that requires attention and care. In today's modern world, we are constantly exposed to a myriad of toxins and pollutants that can overwhelm the body's natural detoxification systems. Therefore, incorporating regular detox practices into our lives can help to mitigate the effects of environmental toxins and promote long-term health and well-being.

Methodology of Dr. Barbara's Herbal Full-Body Detox Program

Dr. Barbara's Herbal Full-Body Detox Program employs a multi-faceted approach to detoxification, addressing various aspects of health and wellness to support the body's natural cleansing processes. The methodology of this program is based on a combination of traditional herbal medicine, nutritional therapy, and lifestyle modifications.

The program begins with an assessment of the individual's health history, current symptoms, and lifestyle factors to determine their unique detoxification needs. This personalized approach allows Dr. Barbara to tailor the program to each individual, taking into account their specific health concerns and goals.

One of the key components of Dr. Barbara's detox program is the use of specific herbs and botanicals that are known for their detoxifying properties. These herbs work synergistically to support liver function, enhance digestion, promote elimination, and neutralize free radicals. Some of the key herbs used in the program include dandelion root, milk thistle, burdock root, and turmeric.

In addition to herbal support, Dr. Barbara's program also emphasizes the importance of dietary modifications to support detoxification. This may include eliminating processed foods, sugar, caffeine, alcohol, and other dietary toxins, and incorporating more whole foods, fruits, vegetables, and clean sources of protein and fats.

Lifestyle modifications are also an integral part of Dr. Barbara's detox program, as stress reduction, adequate sleep, regular exercise, and hydration are essential for supporting the body's natural detoxification processes. Through mindfulness practices, relaxation techniques, and other stress-reducing activities, individuals can enhance the effectiveness of the detox program and promote overall well-being.

Specific Herbs and Botanicals Used in Dr. Barbara's Herbal Full-Body Detox Program

Dr. Barbara's Herbal Full-Body Detox Program utilizes a wide range of herbs and botanicals that are carefully selected for their detoxifying properties and ability to support overall health and vitality. These herbs have been used for centuries in traditional medicine systems around the world and have a long history of safe and effective use.

One of the key herbs used in Dr. Barbara's detox program is dandelion root, which is known for its ability to support liver function and promote bile production. Bile plays a crucial role in the detoxification process, as it helps to transport toxins out of the body through the digestive tract. By supporting bile production, dandelion root helps to enhance the body's natural detoxification pathways.

Milk thistle is another important herb used in Dr. Barbara's detox program, valued for its powerful antioxidant and liver-protective properties. The active compound in milk thistle, silymarin, helps to protect the liver from damage caused by toxins and free radicals, while also stimulating the regeneration of liver cells. This herb is particularly beneficial for individuals with liver conditions or those who have been exposed to environmental toxins.

Burdock root is another key ingredient in Dr. Barbara's detox program, prized for its ability to cleanse the blood and support lymphatic drainage. This herb helps to eliminate toxins from the body by enhancing kidney function and promoting the excretion of waste products through the urine. Burdock root also contains potent antioxidants that help to neutralize free radicals and protect against cellular damage.

Turmeric is a spice that has been used for centuries in traditional medicine for its anti-inflammatory and detoxifying properties. The active compound in turmeric, curcumin, helps to reduce inflammation in the body and support liver function. Turmeric also acts as a potent antioxidant, helping to neutralize free radicals and protect against oxidative stress.

These are just a few examples of the herbs and botanicals used in Dr. Barbara's Herbal Full-Body Detox Program. Each herb is carefully selected for its unique properties and synergistic effects, creating a powerful formula that supports the body's natural detoxification processes and promotes overall health and vitality.

Benefits of Dr. Barbara's Herbal Full-Body Detox Program

The benefits of Dr. Barbara's Herbal Full-Body Detox Program are numerous and far-reaching, encompassing both physical and mental well-being. By supporting the body's natural detoxification processes, this program can help to improve energy levels, enhance digestion, promote weight loss, and boost immunity.

One of the primary benefits of Dr. Barbara's detox program is improved energy and vitality. By eliminating toxins from the body and supporting organ function, individuals often experience a renewed sense of energy and vitality, allowing them to better cope with the demands of daily life.

Improved digestion is another common benefit of Dr. Barbara's detox program. Many individuals experience digestive issues such as bloating, gas, and constipation due to poor dietary choices and environmental toxins. By incorporating herbs and botanicals that support digestive health, this program can help to alleviate these symptoms and promote regularity.

Weight loss is another potential benefit of Dr. Barbara's detox program, as cleansing the body of toxins can help to kickstart the metabolism and promote fat loss. By eliminating processed foods, sugar, and other dietary toxins, individuals may experience weight loss as a natural side effect of the detox process.

In addition to physical benefits, Dr. Barbara's detox program can also have profound effects on mental and emotional well-being. Many individuals report feeling clearer and more focused mentally, as toxins are removed from the body and brain fog lifts. Others experience a greater sense of calm and balance, as stress levels decrease and mood improves.

Overall, Dr. Barbara's Herbal Full-Body Detox Program offers a comprehensive and holistic approach to cleansing and rejuvenating the body. By incorporating herbs, botanicals, dietary modifications, and lifestyle changes, this program supports the body's natural detoxification processes and promotes optimal health and vitality.

CHAPTER TWO

Understanding the Importance of Detoxification for Health and Wellness

Detoxification, often shortened to "detox," has become a popular buzzword in the realm of health and wellness. It refers to the process of eliminating toxins and harmful substances from the body to promote overall health and well-being. While the body has its own natural detoxification mechanisms, the modern world exposes us to an increasing number of environmental toxins, pollutants, and chemicals that can overwhelm these systems. Understanding the importance of detoxification for health and wellness involves exploring how toxins affect the body, the benefits of detoxification, and various methods to support the body's detox processes.

Toxins and Their Impact on Health

Toxins are substances that can harm the body's cells and tissues, leading to a range of health problems. They can come from various sources, including air pollution, pesticides, heavy metals, food additives, alcohol, tobacco smoke, and even stress. Additionally, toxins can be generated internally as byproducts of metabolism or from the breakdown of certain substances in the body.

When toxins accumulate in the body faster than they can be eliminated, they can disrupt normal physiological functions and contribute to the development of chronic diseases. For example, toxins may impair the function of vital organs such as the liver, kidneys, and digestive system, leading to symptoms like fatigue, digestive issues, headaches, skin problems, and weakened immune function. Over time, chronic toxin exposure may increase the risk of conditions such as obesity, diabetes, cardiovascular disease, and cancer.

The Benefits of Detoxification

Given the pervasive nature of toxins in the modern environment, supporting the body's natural detoxification processes is crucial for maintaining optimal health and wellness. Detoxification offers a wide range of potential benefits, including:

1. **Elimination of Toxins**: Detox programs aim to flush toxins from the body, reducing the burden on organs such as the liver, kidneys, and lymphatic system. By eliminating accumulated toxins, detoxification supports the body's natural ability to heal and regenerate.

2. **Improved Energy and Vitality**: Many people report increased energy levels and a sense of vitality after completing a detox program. By removing toxins that can contribute to fatigue and sluggishness, detoxification can leave individuals feeling more energized and rejuvenated.

3. **Enhanced Digestive Health**: Detox diets often emphasize whole, nutrient-dense foods while eliminating processed foods, sugars, and other dietary toxins. This can help to improve digestion, alleviate bloating and gas, and promote regular bowel movements.

4. **Weight Loss Support**: Detox programs may facilitate weight loss by reducing inflammation, balancing hormones, and improving metabolism. By eliminating processed foods and unhealthy habits, individuals may experience weight loss as a natural outcome of the detox process.

5. **Clearer Skin**: Toxins and impurities in the body can contribute to skin problems such as acne, eczema, and dullness. Detoxification supports clearer, healthier skin by promoting the elimination of toxins and reducing inflammation.

6. **Mental Clarity and Focus**: Some individuals experience improved mental clarity, concentration, and mood following a detox program. By removing toxins that can cloud the mind and disrupt neurotransmitter function, detoxification may support cognitive function and emotional well-being.

7. **Immune System Support**: A healthy immune system is essential for defending the body against infections and illnesses. Detoxification helps to remove obstacles to

immune function, allowing the immune system to function optimally and protect against disease.

Methods of Detoxification

There are various methods of detoxification, ranging from dietary changes and lifestyle modifications to specialized detox programs and therapies. Some common approaches to detoxification include:

1. **Healthy Diet**: Eating a diet rich in whole, unprocessed foods, including fruits, vegetables, whole grains, lean proteins, and healthy fats, can support the body's natural detoxification processes. Avoiding processed foods, sugars, alcohol, caffeine, and other dietary toxins can reduce the burden on the body's detox organs.

2. **Hydration**: Drinking an adequate amount of water is essential for flushing toxins from the body and supporting kidney function. Herbal teas, lemon water, and green juices can also support detoxification and hydration.

3. **Exercise**: Regular physical activity promotes circulation, lymphatic drainage, and sweat production, all of which can aid in the elimination of toxins from the body. Activities such as walking, jogging, yoga, and strength training can support detoxification and overall health.

4. **Sauna Therapy**: Sweating is a natural way for the body to eliminate toxins through the skin. Sauna therapy involves sitting in a sauna or steam room to induce sweating and promote detoxification. This can help to remove heavy metals, environmental toxins, and metabolic waste products from the body.

5. **Herbal Supplements**: Certain herbs and botanicals have detoxifying properties and can support the body's natural detoxification processes. Examples include dandelion root, milk thistle, burdock root, turmeric, and cilantro. These herbs can be taken as supplements or incorporated into herbal teas and tinctures.

6. **Colon Cleanses**: Colon cleansing therapies aim to remove waste and toxins from the colon using enemas, colon hydrotherapy, or herbal supplements. While controversial, some people find colon cleanses beneficial for improving digestion and detoxification.

7. **Fasting**: Fasting involves abstaining from food for a certain period, allowing the body to rest and repair while promoting detoxification. Intermittent fasting, juice fasting, and water fasting are some common fasting protocols used for detoxification purposes.

Conclusion

Detoxification is an essential aspect of maintaining health and wellness in today's toxin-laden world. By supporting the body's natural detoxification processes through dietary changes, lifestyle modifications, and specialized detox programs, individuals can reduce the burden of toxins on their bodies and promote optimal health and vitality. Understanding the importance of detoxification for health and wellness involves recognizing the impact of toxins on the body, appreciating the benefits of detoxification, and exploring various methods to support the body's detox processes.

CHAPTER THREE

Dr. Barbara's Philosophy of Herbal Healing and Detoxification

Dr. Barbara's approach to herbal healing and detoxification is deeply rooted in the principles of natural medicine, holistic health, and the profound healing properties of plants. With a background in herbalism and naturopathy, Dr. Barbara has developed a comprehensive philosophy that emphasizes the importance of supporting the body's innate healing abilities, restoring balance, and promoting optimal health through the use of herbal remedies and detoxification protocols.

Holistic Approach to Health and Wellness

Central to Dr. Barbara's philosophy is the understanding that true health and wellness encompass more than just the absence of disease; it involves harmony and balance on physical, mental, emotional, and spiritual levels. Rather than merely treating symptoms, Dr. Barbara believes in addressing the underlying root causes of illness and imbalance to support the body's natural healing processes.

Herbal healing, as practiced by Dr. Barbara, takes a holistic approach that considers the interconnectedness of all aspects of an individual's health and well-being. This approach recognizes the importance of lifestyle factors, diet, emotional well-being, environmental influences, and genetic predispositions in shaping an individual's health status.

Power of Plants in Healing

Dr. Barbara places great emphasis on the healing power of plants and believes that nature provides us with everything we need to support and nourish our bodies. Herbal medicine, which has been practiced for thousands of years across various cultures, harnesses the medicinal properties of plants to promote health and treat a wide range of ailments.

Plants contain a vast array of bioactive compounds, including phytochemicals, antioxidants, vitamins, minerals, and essential oils, which contribute to their therapeutic effects. These natural compounds have been shown to have anti-inflammatory, antimicrobial, antioxidant, analgesic, and detoxifying properties, making them valuable allies in supporting the body's healing processes.

Dr. Barbara's philosophy acknowledges the inherent wisdom of plants and seeks to harness their healing potential through the judicious use of herbal remedies, botanical extracts, and dietary supplements. By working in harmony with nature, Dr. Barbara aims to restore balance and vitality to the body, mind, and spirit.

Detoxification as a Path to Wellness

Detoxification plays a central role in Dr. Barbara's philosophy of herbal healing, as it provides a foundational framework for supporting the body's natural detoxification processes and promoting optimal health and vitality. In today's modern world, we are exposed to an increasing number of environmental toxins, pollutants, and chemicals that can accumulate in the body and disrupt normal physiological functions.

Dr. Barbara believes that regular detoxification is essential for maintaining health and wellness in the face of environmental challenges. By eliminating accumulated toxins, supporting organ function, and promoting the elimination of waste products, detoxification helps to reduce the burden on the body's detoxification organs, such as the liver, kidneys, and lymphatic system.

Dr. Barbara's detoxification protocols incorporate a combination of dietary modifications, herbal supplements, lifestyle changes, and supportive therapies to enhance the body's natural detoxification pathways. By adopting a holistic approach that addresses the root causes of toxicity and supports the body's inherent healing abilities, Dr. Barbara's detox programs aim to promote long-term health, vitality, and resilience.

Individualized Care and Empowerment

Central to Dr. Barbara's philosophy of herbal healing and detoxification is the belief that each individual is unique and deserves personalized care that addresses their specific health needs, goals, and preferences. Dr. Barbara takes the time to listen to her patients, understand their concerns, and develop tailored treatment plans that empower them to take an active role in their health and well-being.

Rather than prescribing one-size-fits-all solutions, Dr. Barbara's approach emphasizes collaboration, education, and empowerment, empowering individuals to make informed choices about their health and lifestyle. By providing personalized guidance, support, and encouragement, Dr. Barbara helps her patients embark on a journey of healing and self-discovery, enabling them to achieve optimal health and vitality.

In conclusion, Dr. Barbara's philosophy of herbal healing and detoxification is founded on the principles of natural medicine, holistic health, and the profound healing power of plants. By embracing a holistic approach that considers the interconnectedness of body, mind, and spirit, Dr. Barbara seeks to restore balance and harmony to the individual, promote optimal health and vitality, and empower her patients to take control of their health and well-being.

CHAPTER FOUR

Preparing Your Body and Mind for the 7-Day Full-Body Detox

Embarking on a 7-day full-body detox journey can be a transformative experience for your health and well-being. However, proper preparation is essential to ensure a smooth and successful detoxification process. In this guide, we'll explore how to prepare your body and mind for a 7-day full-body detox, including dietary adjustments, lifestyle modifications, and mental readiness techniques.

Understanding the Detox Process

Before diving into the preparation phase, it's important to understand what the detox process entails. A full-body detox aims to eliminate toxins and impurities from various organs and systems in the body, including the liver, kidneys, digestive system, lymphatic system, and skin. By supporting these natural detoxification pathways, you can enhance overall health, boost energy levels, and promote well-being.

Setting Clear Intentions

Start by setting clear intentions for your detox journey. What are your goals for the detox? Are you looking to improve energy levels, support digestion, kickstart weight loss, or simply reset your body? By clarifying your intentions, you'll stay focused and motivated throughout the process.

Gradual Dietary Adjustments

Transitioning to a detox-friendly diet before starting the 7-day program can help ease the body into the detox process and minimize potential detox symptoms. Gradually reduce your intake of processed foods, sugars, caffeine, alcohol, and other dietary toxins, while increasing your consumption of whole foods, fruits, vegetables, lean proteins, and healthy fats.

Hydration

Hydration is key to supporting the body's natural detoxification processes. Start increasing your water intake in the days leading up to the detox, aiming for at least 8-10 glasses of water per day. You can also incorporate herbal teas, lemon water, and coconut water for added hydration and detox support.

Supportive Supplements

Consider incorporating supportive supplements into your pre-detox routine to prepare your body for the detox process. This may include herbs and botanicals known for their detoxifying properties, such as dandelion root, milk thistle, burdock root, and turmeric. Consult with a healthcare practitioner to determine which supplements are appropriate for you.

Eliminate Unnecessary Stressors

Reducing stress is essential for optimal detoxification. Identify and eliminate unnecessary stressors from your life in the days leading up to the detox. Practice relaxation techniques such as meditation, deep breathing exercises, yoga, or spending time in nature to promote a calm and centered mindset.

Prepare Your Environment

Create a supportive environment for your detox journey by preparing your kitchen and living space. Stock up on detox-friendly foods, herbal teas, and supplements. Remove temptations such as processed foods, sugary snacks, and alcohol from your home to minimize cravings during the detox.

Mental Readiness

Prepare yourself mentally for the challenges and rewards of the detox process. Remind yourself of your intentions and stay focused on the benefits of cleansing your body and mind. Practice mindfulness, positive affirmations, and visualization techniques to cultivate a positive mindset and enhance resilience.

Seek Support

Consider enlisting the support of friends, family members, or a detox buddy to join you on your journey. Having a support system can provide accountability, encouragement, and motivation throughout the detox process. Share your goals and challenges with your support network and celebrate your successes together.

In conclusion, preparing your body and mind for a 7-day full-body detox involves setting clear intentions, making gradual dietary adjustments, staying hydrated, incorporating supportive supplements, reducing stress, preparing your environment, cultivating a positive mindset, and seeking support from others. By taking these steps, you'll be well-equipped to embark on a successful detox journey and reap the numerous benefits of cleansing your body and revitalizing your health and well-being.

CHAPTER FIVE

Selecting the Right Herbs for Full-Body Cleansing and Healing

Choosing the appropriate herbs for a full-body cleansing and healing regimen is essential for supporting the body's natural detoxification processes and promoting overall wellness. Herbs possess a wide range of therapeutic properties, including detoxification, anti-inflammatory, antioxidant, and immune-boosting effects. In this guide, we'll explore how to select the right herbs for full-body cleansing and healing, considering their specific actions and benefits.

Understanding Your Detox Needs

Before selecting herbs for your full-body cleansing and healing protocol, it's important to understand your detox needs and goals. Consider factors such as your current health status, any specific health concerns or symptoms you're experiencing, and your overall wellness objectives. Are you looking to support liver function, improve digestion, enhance lymphatic drainage, boost immunity, or address inflammation? Identifying your detox needs will help guide your herb selection process.

Key Herbs for Full-Body Cleansing and Healing

1. **Dandelion Root**: Dandelion root is prized for its liver-cleansing properties. It supports liver function by promoting

bile production and flow, aiding in the elimination of toxins from the body. Dandelion root also has diuretic properties, making it beneficial for flushing out excess fluids and reducing water retention.

2. **Milk Thistle**: Milk thistle is one of the most well-known herbs for liver support and detoxification. It contains a compound called silymarin, which helps protect the liver from damage caused by toxins and free radicals. Milk thistle also supports liver regeneration and stimulates the production of glutathione, a powerful antioxidant.

3. **Burdock Root**: Burdock root is a valuable herb for supporting lymphatic drainage and blood purification. It helps remove toxins from the blood and tissues, supports kidney function, and promotes healthy skin. Burdock root is also rich in antioxidants and anti-inflammatory compounds.

4. **Turmeric**: Turmeric is renowned for its anti-inflammatory and antioxidant properties. It contains a compound called curcumin, which helps reduce inflammation, support liver function, and protect against oxidative stress. Turmeric also aids in digestion and promotes overall detoxification.

5. **Ginger**: Ginger is a warming herb that supports digestion, circulation, and detoxification. It helps stimulate the production of digestive enzymes, reduce inflammation in the digestive tract, and promote detoxification through

sweating. Ginger is also beneficial for nausea and gastrointestinal discomfort.

6. **Nettle**: Nettle is a nutrient-rich herb that supports kidney function and urinary tract health. It acts as a diuretic, helping to flush out toxins and excess fluids from the body. Nettle also contains vitamins, minerals, and antioxidants that support overall health and well-being.

7. **Cilantro**: Cilantro is known for its ability to chelate heavy metals and toxins from the body. It binds to heavy metals such as mercury, lead, and aluminum, facilitating their removal from tissues and organs. Cilantro also has anti-inflammatory and digestive benefits.

Choosing High-Quality Herbs

When selecting herbs for full-body cleansing and healing, it's important to choose high-quality, organic herbs from reputable sources. Look for herbs that are free from pesticides, herbicides, and other contaminants. Consider purchasing herbs in their whole, dried form or as standardized extracts to ensure potency and purity.

Consulting with a Healthcare Practitioner

Before starting any herbal detox protocol, it's advisable to consult with a qualified healthcare practitioner, especially if you have any underlying health conditions or are taking medications. A healthcare practitioner can provide personalized guidance and recommendations based on your individual health needs and goals. They can also help ensure that your chosen herbs are safe and appropriate for you.

In conclusion, selecting the right herbs for full-body cleansing and healing involves understanding your detox needs, choosing herbs with specific therapeutic properties, ensuring quality and purity, and consulting with a healthcare practitioner for personalized guidance. By incorporating these key principles, you can create a customized herbal detox protocol that supports your body's natural detoxification processes and promotes optimal health and well-being.

CHAPTER SIX

DR. BARBARA 7-DAY FULL-BODY DETOX PLAN

Creating herbal recipes for each day of a 7-day detox program can add variety, flavor, and therapeutic benefits to your cleansing journey. These recipes incorporate a combination of detoxifying herbs, nutrient-rich ingredients, and cleansing foods to support your body's natural detoxification processes. Here are herbal recipes for each day of the detox program:

Day 1: Detoxifying Green Smoothie

Ingredients:

- 1 cup spinach or kale (fresh or frozen)

- 1/2 cucumber, peeled and chopped

- 1/2 green apple, cored and chopped

- 1 tablespoon fresh cilantro leaves

- 1 tablespoon fresh parsley leaves

- 1 teaspoon grated ginger

- Juice of 1/2 lemon

- 1 cup coconut water or filtered water

- Optional: 1 tablespoon chia seeds or flaxseeds

Instructions:

1. Combine all ingredients in a blender.

2. Blend until smooth and creamy.

3. Pour into a glass and enjoy immediately.

Day 2: Turmeric Detox Tea

Ingredients:

- 1 teaspoon ground turmeric

- 1/2 teaspoon ground cinnamon

- 1/4 teaspoon ground ginger

- Pinch of black pepper (to enhance turmeric absorption)

- 1 tablespoon raw honey or maple syrup (optional)

- 2 cups filtered water

- Juice of 1/2 lemon

Instructions:

1. In a small saucepan, bring the water to a boil.

2. Add turmeric, cinnamon, ginger, and black pepper to the boiling water.

3. Reduce heat and simmer for 5-10 minutes.

4. Remove from heat and stir in honey or maple syrup (if using) and lemon juice.

5. Strain the tea into mugs and enjoy warm.

Day 3: Cleansing Detox Salad

Ingredients:

- 2 cups mixed greens (spinach, arugula, kale)

- 1/2 cup grated carrots

- 1/2 cup grated beets

- 1/4 cup thinly sliced red cabbage

- 1/4 cup chopped fresh parsley

- 1/4 cup pumpkin seeds or sunflower seeds

- Dressing: 2 tablespoons extra virgin olive oil, 1 tablespoon apple cider vinegar, 1 teaspoon Dijon mustard, salt, and pepper to taste

Instructions:

1. In a large mixing bowl, combine mixed greens, grated carrots, grated beets, red cabbage, parsley, and seeds.

2. In a small bowl, whisk together the dressing ingredients until well combined.

3. Pour the dressing over the salad and toss until evenly coated.

4. Serve immediately or refrigerate until ready to serve.

Day 4: Detoxifying Herbal Soup

Ingredients:

- 1 tablespoon olive oil or coconut oil

- 1 onion, chopped

- 2 cloves garlic, minced

- 2 carrots, diced

- 2 celery stalks, diced

- 1 zucchini, diced

- 4 cups vegetable broth

- 1 cup chopped kale or spinach

- 1 tablespoon chopped fresh thyme

- 1 tablespoon chopped fresh parsley

- Salt and pepper to taste

Instructions:

1. Heat oil in a large pot over medium heat. Add onion and garlic and sauté until softened.

2. Add carrots, celery, and zucchini to the pot and cook for another 5 minutes.

3. Pour in vegetable broth and bring to a simmer.

4. Add kale or spinach, thyme, and parsley to the pot and simmer for 10-15 minutes until vegetables are tender.

5. Season with salt and pepper to taste.

6. Ladle soup into bowls and serve hot.

Day 5: Herbal Detox Water

Ingredients:

- 1 lemon, thinly sliced

- 1/2 cucumber, thinly sliced

- 1 inch fresh ginger, thinly sliced

- Handful of fresh mint leaves

- 2-3 cups filtered water

- Ice cubes (optional)

Instructions:

1. In a large pitcher, combine lemon slices, cucumber slices, ginger slices, and mint leaves.

2. Fill the pitcher with filtered water.

3. Refrigerate for at least 1 hour to allow the flavors to infuse.

4. Serve over ice cubes, if desired.

Day 6: Detoxifying Herbal Tea Blend

Ingredients:

- 1 tablespoon dried dandelion root

- 1 tablespoon dried burdock root

- 1 tablespoon dried nettle leaf

- 1 tablespoon dried cleavers

- 1 tablespoon dried peppermint leaf

- 4 cups filtered water

- Honey or maple syrup (optional, for sweetness)

Instructions:

1. In a medium saucepan, bring water to a boil.

2. Add dried herbs to the boiling water.

3. Reduce heat and simmer for 10-15 minutes.

4. Remove from heat and let the tea steep for an additional 5 minutes.

5. Strain the tea into cups and sweeten with honey or maple syrup if desired.

6. Enjoy warm or chilled.

Day 7: Detoxifying Herbal Broth

Ingredients:

- 8 cups water
- 1 onion, chopped
- 2 carrots, chopped
- 2 celery stalks, chopped
- 1 cup chopped mushrooms
- 2 cloves garlic, minced
- 1-inch piece of ginger, grated
- 1 tablespoon dried thyme
- 1 tablespoon dried rosemary
- 1 tablespoon dried sage
- Salt and pepper to taste

Instructions:

1. In a large pot, bring water to a boil.
2. Add onion, carrots, celery, mushrooms, garlic, and ginger to the pot.
3. Stir in dried herbs and season with salt and pepper.

4. Reduce heat and simmer for 1-2 hours.

5. Strain the broth into a large bowl or container.

6. Serve the herbal broth hot as a comforting drink or use it as a base for soups and stews.

These herbal recipes provide a nourishing and supportive framework for your 7-day detox program, incorporating a variety of detoxifying herbs and ingredients to promote cleansing, healing, and rejuvenation of the body and mind. Enjoy these recipes as part of your detox journey and feel the transformative effects of herbal healing and nourishment.

CHAPTER SEVEN

Incorporating herbal teas and supplements into your detoxification regimen

Incorporating herbal teas and supplements into your detoxification regimen can enhance the effectiveness of your cleanse by providing additional support to your body's natural detoxification pathways. Herbal teas contain potent medicinal compounds that can promote detoxification, while supplements offer concentrated doses of specific nutrients and herbs to target detoxification processes. Here's how to incorporate herbal teas and supplements for enhanced detoxification:

Herbal Teas for Detoxification

1. **Dandelion Root Tea**: Dandelion root is known for its liver-cleansing properties. Drinking dandelion root tea can support liver function, aid digestion, and promote the elimination of toxins from the body.

2. **Milk Thistle Tea**: Milk thistle is a powerful herb for liver support and detoxification. Milk thistle tea contains silymarin, a compound that protects the liver from damage and promotes liver regeneration.

3. **Nettle Tea**: Nettle tea is rich in vitamins, minerals, and antioxidants that support detoxification and kidney function.

It acts as a diuretic, helping to flush out toxins and excess fluids from the body.

4. **Ginger Tea**: Ginger tea supports digestion, circulation, and detoxification. It helps stimulate the production of digestive enzymes, reduce inflammation, and promote sweating, which aids in the elimination of toxins.

5. **Turmeric Tea**: Turmeric tea contains curcumin, a powerful antioxidant and anti-inflammatory compound that supports liver function and detoxification. Drinking turmeric tea can help reduce inflammation and promote overall detoxification.

Supplements for Detoxification

1. **Milk Thistle Extract**: Milk thistle extract is available in supplement form and provides a concentrated dose of silymarin, the active compound in milk thistle. Taking milk thistle extract can support liver health, protect against liver damage, and enhance detoxification.

2. **N-Acetylcysteine (NAC)**: NAC is a precursor to glutathione, a powerful antioxidant and detoxifier produced by the liver. Taking NAC supplements can boost glutathione levels, support liver function, and enhance detoxification.

3. **Activated Charcoal**: Activated charcoal supplements can bind to toxins and chemicals in the gut, preventing their

absorption into the bloodstream and facilitating their elimination from the body. Taking activated charcoal supplements can help reduce bloating, gas, and detoxification symptoms.

4. **Chlorella**: Chlorella is a type of algae rich in chlorophyll, vitamins, minerals, and antioxidants. Taking chlorella supplements can support detoxification by binding to heavy metals and toxins in the body and promoting their elimination.

5. **Probiotics**: Probiotic supplements contain beneficial bacteria that support gut health and digestion. Taking probiotics can help maintain a healthy balance of gut flora, which is essential for detoxification and overall health.

Incorporating Herbal Teas and Supplements into Your Detox Routine

1. **Morning Ritual**: Start your day with a cup of herbal tea, such as dandelion root or ginger tea, to support liver function and digestion. Take your supplements with breakfast to kickstart your detoxification process.

2. **Throughout the Day**: Sip on herbal teas throughout the day to stay hydrated and support detoxification. Rotate between different teas, such as milk thistle, nettle, and turmeric, to reap their unique benefits.

3. **Before Bed**: Wind down in the evening with a calming herbal tea, such as chamomile or peppermint, to promote relaxation and digestion. Take any evening supplements, such as activated charcoal or probiotics, to support overnight detoxification.

4. **Consistency is Key**: Incorporate herbal teas and supplements into your daily routine consistently throughout your detox program to maximize their effectiveness. Remember to follow the recommended dosage guidelines for supplements and consult with a healthcare practitioner if you have any underlying health conditions or concerns.

By incorporating herbal teas and supplements into your detoxification regimen, you can support your body's natural detoxification processes, enhance liver function, promote digestion, and optimize overall health and well-being. Experiment with different teas and supplements to find what works best for you, and enjoy the rejuvenating benefits of enhanced detoxification.

CHAPTER EIGHT

Managing detox symptoms and supporting your body's natural processes

Managing detox symptoms and supporting your body's natural processes are essential aspects of a successful detoxification journey. While detoxing can lead to temporary discomfort as toxins are released from the body, there are several strategies you can employ to minimize symptoms and promote overall well-being. Here's how to manage detox symptoms and support your body's natural processes during a detox program:

Hydration:

1. **Drink Plenty of Water**: Staying hydrated is crucial for supporting detoxification and flushing out toxins from the body. Aim to drink at least 8-10 glasses of water per day, or more if you're sweating heavily or experiencing detox symptoms like headaches or fatigue.

Nutrient-Rich Diet: 2. Eat Whole Foods: Focus on consuming a nutrient-dense diet rich in fruits, vegetables, whole grains, lean proteins, and healthy fats. These foods provide essential vitamins, minerals, antioxidants, and fiber to support detoxification and overall health.

Herbal Support: 3. Herbal Teas: Drink herbal teas known for their detoxifying properties, such as dandelion root, milk thistle, nettle, ginger, and turmeric. These teas can support liver function, aid digestion, and promote the elimination of toxins from the body.

Gentle Exercise: 4. **Engage in Light Exercise**: Gentle exercise, such as walking, yoga, stretching, or swimming, can help stimulate circulation, promote lymphatic drainage, and support the body's natural detoxification processes. Avoid intense or strenuous exercise during a detox program, as your body may be more sensitive to exertion.

Rest and Relaxation: 5. **Prioritize Sleep**: Get plenty of restorative sleep to support your body's detoxification efforts and overall well-being. Aim for 7-9 hours of quality sleep per night, and create a relaxing bedtime routine to promote deep, restful sleep.

Supportive Therapies: 6. **Dry Brushing**: Dry brushing the skin stimulates the lymphatic system, promotes circulation, and helps eliminate toxins through the skin. Use a natural-bristle brush to gently exfoliate the skin in long, sweeping motions towards the heart before showering.

Mind-Body Practices: 7. **Practice Stress Reduction Techniques**: Chronic stress can impede the body's detoxification processes and exacerbate detox symptoms. Incorporate stress reduction techniques such as meditation, deep breathing exercises, mindfulness, or journaling to promote relaxation and emotional well-being.

Listen to Your Body: 8. **Pay Attention to Your Body's Signals**: Listen to your body and honor its needs during the detox process. If you're experiencing severe detox symptoms or discomfort, consider scaling back on the intensity of your detox program or seeking guidance from a healthcare practitioner.

Gradual Transition: 9. **Ease Into and Out of Detox**: Gradually transition into and out of your detox program to minimize potential detox symptoms. Start by reducing your intake of processed foods, caffeine, alcohol, and sugar before beginning the detox, and gradually reintroduce these foods after completing the program.

Consult with a Healthcare Practitioner: 10. **Seek Professional Guidance**: If you have any underlying health conditions or concerns, or if you're unsure about how to safely detoxify, consult with a qualified healthcare practitioner before starting a detox program. They can provide personalized guidance and recommendations based on your individual health needs and goals.

By implementing these strategies, you can effectively manage detox symptoms, support your body's natural detoxification processes, and optimize your overall health and well-being during a detox program. Remember to listen to your body, prioritize self-care, and seek professional guidance as needed to ensure a safe and successful detoxification journey.

CHAPTER NINE

Mindfulness and self-care practices

Mindfulness and self-care practices play a crucial role in supporting your well-being during a detox week. These practices can help you stay grounded, manage stress, and cultivate a positive mindset throughout your detox journey. Here are some mindfulness and self-care practices to incorporate into your detox week:

Daily Meditation:

1. **Mindful Breathing**: Take a few minutes each day to practice mindful breathing. Sit comfortably, close your eyes, and focus on your breath as it flows in and out of your body. Notice the sensations of each inhale and exhale, and gently bring your attention back to your breath whenever your mind wanders.

Body Awareness: 2. Body Scan Meditation: Practice a body scan meditation to cultivate awareness of physical sensations in your body. Start at your feet and slowly move your attention upwards, scanning each part of your body for any tension, discomfort, or areas of relaxation. Notice any sensations without judgment and allow them to be as they are.

Gratitude Practice: 3. Gratitude Journaling: Take a few moments each day to write down three things you're grateful for. Reflect on the positive aspects of your life, no matter how small, and express gratitude for them. Cultivating a sense of gratitude can help shift your focus away from detox symptoms and challenges towards the blessings in your life.

Nature Connection: 4. **Outdoor Walks**: Spend time in nature by going for a walk in a nearby park, forest, or natural setting. Notice the sights, sounds, and sensations of the natural world around you. Connecting with nature can help reduce stress, improve mood, and promote a sense of well-being.

Nourishing Activities: 5. **Healthy Cooking**: Prepare nourishing meals using whole, detox-friendly ingredients. Engage all your senses as you chop, cook, and savor each bite. Cooking can be a mindful activity that fosters a deeper connection with the food you eat and promotes overall well-being.

Self-Compassion: 6. **Self-Compassion Meditation**: Practice self-compassion by offering yourself kindness, understanding, and support during the detox week. Use phrases such as "May I be kind to myself" or "May I embrace myself with love and acceptance" as you cultivate a compassionate attitude towards yourself and your experiences.

Digital Detox: 7. **Unplug**: Take breaks from screens and digital devices to reduce mental clutter and overwhelm. Disconnect from social media, email, and other digital distractions for periods of time each day. Instead, engage in activities that nourish your soul, such as reading, spending time with loved ones, or pursuing hobbies.

Relaxation Techniques: 8. **Progressive Muscle Relaxation**: Practice progressive muscle relaxation to release tension and promote relaxation throughout your body. Start by tensing and then releasing each muscle group, starting from your toes and working your way up to your head.

Mindful Movement: 9. **Yoga or Tai Chi**: Engage in gentle movement practices such as yoga or Tai Chi to promote relaxation, flexibility, and body awareness. Focus on the sensations of movement, breath, and presence in the moment as you flow through each posture or movement sequence.

Social Connection: 10. **Reach Out**: Connect with supportive friends, family members, or fellow detox participants for encouragement, inspiration, and accountability. Share your experiences, challenges, and victories with others who understand and support your journey.

By incorporating these mindfulness and self-care practices into your detox week, you can nurture your body, mind, and spirit, and enhance your overall well-being. Remember to prioritize self-care, listen to your body's needs, and approach the detox process with kindness, curiosity, and compassion.

CHAPTER TEN

Post-detox maintenance

Post-detox maintenance is essential for sustaining the results of your detox program and continuing your wellness journey in the long term. After completing a detox, it's important to transition back to a balanced and sustainable lifestyle that supports your health and well-being. Here are some tips for post-detox maintenance:

1. Gradual Reintroduction of Foods:

- After completing your detox, gradually reintroduce foods that were restricted during the detox period, such as caffeine, alcohol, processed foods, and sugar. Pay attention to how your body responds to these foods and make mindful choices based on how they make you feel.

2. Focus on Whole Foods:

- Continue to prioritize whole, nutrient-rich foods in your diet, such as fruits, vegetables, whole grains, lean proteins, and healthy fats. These foods provide essential vitamins, minerals, antioxidants, and fiber to support overall health and well-being.

3. Hydration:

- Maintain adequate hydration by drinking plenty of water throughout the day. Aim for at least 8-10 glasses of water per day to support detoxification, hydration, and overall health.

4. Mindful Eating:

- Practice mindful eating by paying attention to your hunger and fullness cues, eating slowly, and savoring each bite. Be present and engaged with your food, and cultivate awareness of how different foods make you feel physically, mentally, and emotionally.

5. Regular Physical Activity:

- Stay active by incorporating regular exercise into your routine. Choose activities that you enjoy, such as walking, jogging, cycling, yoga, or strength training, and aim for at least 30 minutes of moderate-intensity exercise most days of the week.

6. Stress Management:

- Continue to prioritize stress management techniques such as meditation, deep breathing exercises, yoga, mindfulness, or spending time in nature. Manage stress effectively to support overall health, well-being, and resilience.

7. Quality Sleep:

- Prioritize restorative sleep by maintaining a consistent sleep schedule, creating a relaxing bedtime routine, and optimizing your sleep environment. Aim for 7-9 hours of quality sleep per night to support detoxification, recovery, and overall health.

8. Regular Detox Practices:

- Incorporate regular detox practices into your routine to support ongoing cleansing and rejuvenation of your body and mind. This could include periodic juice cleanses, herbal detox protocols, sauna sessions, or intermittent fasting.

9. Mindfulness and Self-Care:

- Continue to prioritize mindfulness and self-care practices to nurture your body, mind, and spirit. Engage in activities that bring you joy, relaxation, and fulfillment, and make time for self-reflection, creativity, and connection with others.

10. Listen to Your Body:

- Tune in to your body's signals and honor its needs as you navigate post-detox maintenance. Pay attention to how different foods, activities, and lifestyle choices affect your energy levels, mood, digestion, and overall well-being.

11. Seek Support:

- Surround yourself with supportive friends, family members, or healthcare practitioners who can offer encouragement, guidance, and accountability as you continue your wellness journey. Share your goals, challenges, and successes with others who understand and support your efforts.

By implementing these post-detox maintenance tips, you can sustain the results of your detox program, optimize your health and well-being, and continue your journey towards lasting wellness and vitality. Remember that wellness is a lifelong journey, and small, consistent actions can lead to significant and sustainable improvements in your health and quality of life.

BONUS: SOME HOLISTIC REMEDIES TO KNOW

Goldenseal:

Definition: Goldenseal, scientifically known as Hydrastis canadensis, is a perennial herb native to North America. It has a long history of use in traditional Native American medicine and later in folk medicine for its potential health benefits.

Ingredients: Goldenseal root contains various bioactive compounds, including alkaloids (such as berberine and hydrastine), flavonoids, and volatile oils. These compounds are believed to contribute to the herb's medicinal properties, including its potential as an antimicrobial, anti-inflammatory, and immune enhancer.

How to Prepare: Goldenseal is typically consumed as an herbal tea, tincture, or in supplement form (such as capsules or tablets). To make tea, dried goldenseal root or leaves are steeped in hot water for several minutes before being strained and consumed.

Dosage: The appropriate dosage of goldenseal can vary depending on factors such as age, health status, and the specific preparation being used. It's important to follow the recommended dosage on the product label or consult with a qualified herbalist or healthcare professional for personalized guidance.

How to Use: Goldenseal tea, tincture, or supplements are typically taken orally. It's often used to support immune function, promote digestive health, and soothe inflammation.

Side Effects: Goldenseal is generally considered safe for most people when used in moderate amounts. However, some individuals may experience mild side effects such as gastrointestinal upset or allergic reactions. It may also interact with certain medications or have adverse effects in individuals with certain health conditions, such as high blood pressure or pregnancy. It's important to use goldenseal under the guidance of a healthcare professional and to discontinue use if any adverse effects occur.

Bio Ferro Tonic:

Definition: Bio Ferro Tonic is a dietary supplement primarily composed of herbs and minerals. It's often marketed as a natural way to support overall health, particularly by promoting blood health and circulation.

Ingredients: Typical ingredients in Bio Ferro Tonic may include a blend of herbs such as burdock root, yellow dock root, sarsaparilla root, and cascara sagrada bark, along with minerals like iron and potassium phosphate.

How to Prepare: Bio Ferro Tonic usually comes in liquid form and is typically taken orally. It's important to follow the instructions on the product label for dosage and administration.

Dosage: The dosage can vary depending on the specific product and individual needs. It's crucial to consult with a healthcare professional or follow the recommended dosage on the product label to avoid potential side effects.

How to Use: Bio Ferro Tonic is often taken by adding the recommended dosage to water or juice and consuming it orally. It's important to shake the bottle well before use and store it according to the manufacturer's instructions.

Side Effects: While Bio Ferro Tonic is generally considered safe when used as directed, some individuals may experience side effects such as digestive discomfort, allergic reactions, or interactions with medications. It's essential to consult with a healthcare provider before starting any new supplement regimen, especially if you have underlying health conditions or are taking medications.

Bladderwrack:

Definition: Bladderwrack is a type of seaweed or marine algae commonly used in traditional medicine and as a dietary supplement. It's known for its potential health benefits, particularly related to thyroid health and weight management.

Ingredients: Bladderwrack contains various nutrients, including iodine, vitamins, minerals, and antioxidants. The primary active components are iodine and fucoidan, a type of carbohydrate found in brown seaweeds.

How to Prepare: Bladderwrack supplements are available in various forms, including capsules, powders, and liquid extracts. They can be taken orally with water or added to smoothies and other beverages.

Dosage: The appropriate dosage of bladderwrack can vary based on factors such as age, health status, and the specific product being used. It's essential to follow the recommended dosage on the product label or consult with a healthcare professional for personalized guidance.

How to Use: Bladderwrack supplements are typically taken orally, either with water or mixed into food or beverages. It's important to follow the instructions on the product label and avoid exceeding the recommended dosage.

Side Effects: While bladderwrack is generally considered safe for most people when used in moderation, excessive intake of iodine from bladderwrack supplements can cause thyroid dysfunction and other adverse effects. Individuals with thyroid disorders, iodine sensitivity, or certain medical conditions should exercise caution and consult with a healthcare provider before using bladderwrack supplements. Common side effects may include digestive upset, allergic reactions, or interactions with medications.

Blood Purifier:

Definition: Blood purifiers are herbal remedies or dietary supplements believed to cleanse or detoxify the blood, often promoting overall health and well-being. They are thought to support the body's natural detoxification processes and improve blood circulation.

Ingredients: Blood purifiers may contain a variety of herbs and botanical extracts known for their purported cleansing and detoxifying properties. Common ingredients include burdock root, red clover, dandelion root, and yellow dock root, among others.

How to Prepare: Blood purifiers are typically available in various forms, including capsules, tablets, powders, and liquid extracts. They are usually taken orally with water or juice, following the recommended dosage on the product label.

Dosage: The dosage of blood purifiers can vary depending on the specific product and individual needs. It's important to adhere to the recommended dosage on the product label or consult with a healthcare professional for personalized guidance.

How to Use: Blood purifiers are typically taken orally, either with water or mixed into beverages. They are often used as part of a detoxification regimen or to support overall health and vitality.

Side Effects: While blood purifiers are generally considered safe for most people when used as directed, some individuals may experience side effects such as digestive discomfort, allergic reactions, or interactions with medications. It's important to consult with a healthcare provider before starting any new supplement regimen, especially if you have underlying health conditions or are taking medications.

Blue Vervain:

Definition: Blue vervain, also known as Verbena hastata, is a perennial herb native to North America. It has been used in traditional medicine for centuries to treat various ailments, including anxiety, insomnia, and digestive issues.

Ingredients: Blue vervain contains several active compounds, including aucubin, verbenalin, and volatile oils. These compounds are believed to contribute to the herb's medicinal properties.

How to Prepare: Blue vervain is typically consumed as a tea or tincture. To make tea, dried blue vervain leaves and flowers are steeped in hot water for several minutes before being strained and consumed. Tinctures are prepared by steeping the herb in alcohol or vinegar to extract its active compounds.

Dosage: The appropriate dosage of blue vervain can vary depending on factors such as age, health status, and the specific preparation being used. It's important to follow the recommended dosage on the product label or consult with a qualified herbalist or healthcare professional for personalized guidance.

How to Use: Blue vervain tea or tincture is typically taken orally. It can be consumed on its own or mixed with honey or other herbal teas for added flavor.

Side Effects: While blue vervain is generally considered safe for most people when used in moderation, excessive intake may cause digestive upset or allergic reactions in some individuals. Pregnant or breastfeeding women should avoid blue vervain due to its potential to stimulate uterine contractions. As with any herbal remedy, it's important to consult with a healthcare provider before using blue vervain, especially if you have underlying health conditions or are taking medications.

Bromide Plus Powder:

Definition: Bromide Plus Powder is a dietary supplement formulated to support thyroid health and promote overall well-being. It typically contains a blend of herbs and minerals that are believed to have beneficial effects on thyroid function.

Ingredients: Bromide Plus Powder often contains a combination of herbs such as bladderwrack, sea moss, and burdock root, along with minerals like iodine and potassium phosphate. These ingredients are thought to support thyroid function and maintain optimal iodine levels in the body.

How to Prepare: Bromide Plus Powder is usually mixed with water or juice to create a drinkable solution. It's important to follow the instructions on the product label for dosage and preparation.

Dosage: The dosage of Bromide Plus Powder can vary depending on the specific product and individual needs. It's crucial to consult with a healthcare professional or follow the recommended dosage on the product label to avoid potential side effects.

How to Use: Bromide Plus Powder is typically taken orally by mixing the recommended dosage with water or juice. It's important to shake or stir the mixture well before consuming it to ensure even distribution of the ingredients.

Side Effects: While Bromide Plus Powder is generally considered safe when used as directed, some individuals may experience side effects such as digestive discomfort or allergic reactions to certain ingredients. It's essential to consult with a healthcare provider before starting any new supplement regimen, especially if you have underlying health conditions or are taking medications.

Bugleweed:

Definition: Bugleweed, also known as Lycopusvirginicus, is a perennial herb native to North America and Europe. It has been used in traditional medicine to treat various conditions, including hyperthyroidism, anxiety, and insomnia.

Ingredients: Bugleweed contains several active compounds, including lithospermic acid, phenolic acids, and flavonoids. These compounds are believed to contribute to the herb's medicinal properties, particularly its ability to regulate thyroid function.

How to Prepare: Bugleweed is commonly consumed as a tea or tincture. To make tea, dried bugleweed leaves and flowers are steeped in hot water for several minutes before being strained and consumed. Tinctures are prepared by steeping the herb in alcohol or vinegar to extract its active compounds.

Dosage: The appropriate dosage of bugleweed can vary depending on factors such as age, health status, and the specific preparation being used. It's important to follow the recommended dosage on the product label or consult with a qualified herbalist or healthcare professional for personalized guidance.

How to Use: Bugleweed tea or tincture is typically taken orally. It can be consumed on its own or mixed with honey or other herbal teas for added flavor.

Side Effects: While bugleweed is generally considered safe for most people when used in moderation, excessive intake may cause digestive upset or allergic reactions in some individuals. Pregnant or breastfeeding women should avoid bugleweed due to its potential to stimulate uterine contractions. As with any herbal remedy, it's important to consult with a healthcare provider before using bugleweed, especially if you have underlying health conditions or are taking medications.

Burdock:

Definition: Burdock, scientifically known as Arctium lappa, is a biennial plant native to Europe and Asia but now found worldwide. It's part of the Asteraceae family and has been used for centuries in traditional medicine and culinary practices.

Ingredients: Burdock contains various nutrients, including carbohydrates, fiber, vitamins (such as vitamin B6, folate, and vitamin C), and minerals (including potassium, magnesium, and manganese). It also contains active compounds such as polyphenols and volatile oils.

How to Prepare: Burdock can be prepared and consumed in various ways. The roots, leaves, and seeds are all utilized for different purposes. The root is commonly used in cooking, herbal teas, tinctures, and supplements, while the leaves and seeds are sometimes used in herbal preparations.

Dosage: The appropriate dosage of burdock root can vary depending on the specific form and intended use. For culinary purposes, there are no strict dosage guidelines, but for supplements or herbal remedies, it's essential to follow the recommended dosage on the product label or consult with a healthcare professional.

How to Use: Burdock root can be used in cooking by peeling, slicing, and adding it to soups, stews, stir-fries, or salads. It can also be brewed into a tea or used to make tinctures or extracts for medicinal purposes. Some people may also take burdock root supplements in capsule or powder form.

Side Effects: While burdock is generally considered safe for most people when consumed in moderate amounts, some individuals may experience allergic reactions or digestive upset. Additionally, burdock may interact with certain medications or have adverse effects in individuals with certain health conditions, such as diabetes or allergies to plants in the Asteraceae family. It's important to consult with a healthcare provider before using burdock, especially if you have underlying health conditions or are taking medications.

Cascara Sagrada:

Definition: Cascara Sagrada, scientifically known as Rhamnus purshiana, is a species of buckthorn native to western North

America. It has been used traditionally as a laxative and to promote bowel regularity.

Ingredients: The primary active ingredients in cascara sagrada are anthraquinone glycosides, particularly cascarosides A and B. These compounds stimulate peristalsis in the colon, leading to increased bowel movements.

How to Prepare: Cascara sagrada is typically prepared as an herbal tea, tincture, or capsule. To make tea, dried cascara sagrada bark is steeped in hot water for several minutes before being strained and consumed. Tinctures are prepared by steeping the bark in alcohol to extract its active compounds.

Dosage: The appropriate dosage of cascara sagrada can vary depending on the specific preparation and intended use. It's important to follow the recommended dosage on the product label or consult with a healthcare professional for personalized guidance.

How to Use: Cascara sagrada tea or tincture is typically taken orally. It's important to start with a low dose and gradually increase if needed to avoid potential side effects such as cramping or diarrhea.

Side Effects: Cascara sagrada is considered safe for short-term use when used as directed. However, long-term or excessive use may lead to dependence, electrolyte imbalance, or dehydration.

It may also interact with certain medications or have adverse effects in individuals with certain health conditions. It's important to use cascara sagrada under the guidance of a healthcare professional and to discontinue use if any adverse effects occur.

Cocolmeca:

Definition: Cocolmeca, also known as Smilax ornata or sarsaparilla, is a flowering vine native to Mexico and Central America. It has been used traditionally in Mexican and Central American folk medicine for its purported medicinal properties.

Ingredients: Cocolmeca contains various bioactive compounds, including saponins, flavonoids, and plant sterols. These compounds are believed to contribute to the herb's medicinal properties, including its potential as a diuretic, blood purifier, and anti-inflammatory agent.

How to Prepare: Cocolmeca is commonly prepared and consumed as an herbal tea or decoction. To make tea, dried cocolmeca roots or leaves are steeped in hot water for several minutes before being strained and consumed. Decoctions involve boiling the roots or leaves in water to extract their active compounds.

Dosage: The appropriate dosage of cocolmeca can vary depending on factors such as age, health status, and the specific preparation being used. It's important to follow the recommended dosage on the product label or consult with a qualified herbalist or healthcare professional for personalized guidance.

How to Use: Cocolmeca tea or decoction is typically taken orally. It can also be used topically for certain skin conditions. It's important to use cocolmeca products as directed and to discontinue use if any adverse effects occur.

Side Effects: Cocolmeca is generally considered safe for most people when used in moderate amounts. However, excessive intake may lead to digestive upset or other adverse effects. It may also interact with certain medications or have adverse effects in individuals with certain health conditions. It's important to use cocolmeca under the guidance of a healthcare professional and to discontinue use if any adverse effects occur.

Contribo:

Definition: Contribo, also known as Aristolochiatrilobata, is a vine native to the Caribbean and Central America. It has been used traditionally in folk medicine for various purposes, including as a remedy for digestive issues, inflammation, and pain relief.

Ingredients: Contribo contains several bioactive compounds, including aristolochic acids, flavonoids, and alkaloids. These compounds are believed to contribute to the herb's medicinal properties, including its potential as an anti-inflammatory and analgesic agent.

How to Prepare: Contribo is typically prepared and consumed as an herbal tea or decoction. To make tea, dried contribo leaves or stems are steeped in hot water for several minutes before being strained and consumed. Decoctions involve boiling the leaves or stems in water to extract their active compounds.

Dosage: The appropriate dosage of contribo can vary depending on factors such as age, health status, and the specific preparation being used. It's important to follow the recommended dosage on the product label or consult with a qualified herbalist or healthcare professional for personalized guidance.

How to Use: Contribo tea or decoction is typically taken orally. It's important to use contribo products as directed and to discontinue use if any adverse effects occur.

Side Effects: Contribo contains aristolochic acids, which have been associated with serious adverse effects, including kidney damage and cancer. Due to these safety concerns, the use of contribo is highly discouraged, and it's important to avoid products containing aristolochic acids. Individuals should seek alternative remedies for their health needs.

Dandelion Root:

Definition: Dandelion, scientifically known as Taraxacum officinale, is a common flowering plant found worldwide. While often considered a pesky weed, dandelion has a long history of use in traditional medicine for its various health benefits.

Ingredients: Dandelion root contains several bioactive compounds, including sesquiterpene lactones, triterpenes, flavonoids, and polysaccharides. These compounds are believed to contribute to the herb's medicinal properties, including its potential as a diuretic, digestive aid, and liver tonic.

How to Prepare: Dandelion root can be prepared and consumed in various forms, including teas, tinctures, capsules, and extracts. To make tea, dried dandelion root is steeped in hot water for several minutes before being strained and consumed. Tinctures are prepared by steeping the root in alcohol or vinegar to extract its active compounds.

Dosage: The appropriate dosage of dandelion root can vary depending on factors such as age, health status, and the specific preparation being used. It's important to follow the recommended dosage on the product label or consult with a qualified herbalist or healthcare professional for personalized guidance.

How to Use: Dandelion root tea, tincture, or capsules are typically taken orally. It's important to use dandelion root products as directed and to discontinue use if any adverse effects occur.

Side Effects: Dandelion root is generally considered safe for most people when used in moderate amounts. However, some individuals may experience allergic reactions or digestive upset. It may also interact with certain medications or have adverse effects in individuals with certain health conditions. It's important to use dandelion root under the guidance of a healthcare professional and to discontinue use if any adverse effects occur.

Green Food Plus:

Definition: Green Food Plus is a dietary supplement formulated to provide a concentrated source of nutrients derived from various green plants. It's designed to support overall health and well-being by delivering essential vitamins, minerals, antioxidants, and phytonutrients.

Ingredients: Green Food Plus typically contains a blend of powdered green vegetables, grasses, algae, and other plant-based ingredients. Common ingredients may include wheatgrass, barley grass, spirulina, chlorella, alfalfa, kale, spinach, and broccoli, among others.

How to Prepare: Green Food Plus is usually available in powder form and can be mixed with water, juice, or smoothies. It's important to follow the recommended dosage on the product label and to consume it as part of a balanced diet.

Dosage: The appropriate dosage of Green Food Plus can vary depending on the specific product and individual needs. It's important to follow the recommended dosage on the product label or consult with a healthcare professional for personalized guidance.

How to Use: Green Food Plus powder is typically mixed with water, juice, or smoothies and consumed orally. It's often taken once or twice daily, preferably with meals, to maximize nutrient absorption.

Side Effects: Green Food Plus is generally considered safe for most people when used as directed. However, some individuals may experience digestive upset or allergic reactions to certain ingredients. It's important to consult with a healthcare provider before starting any new supplement regimen, especially if you have underlying health conditions or are taking medications.

Guaco:

Definition: Guaco, also known as Mikania cordata or Mikania glomerata, is a medicinal plant native to Central and South America. It has a long history of use in traditional medicine for its potential therapeutic properties.

Ingredients: Guaco contains several bioactive compounds, including coumarins, flavonoids, tannins, and saponins. These compounds are believed to contribute to the herb's medicinal properties, including its potential as an expectorant, anti-inflammatory, and antispasmodic agent.

How to Prepare: Guaco is typically prepared and consumed as an herbal tea or infusion. To make tea, dried guaco leaves are steeped in hot water for several minutes before being strained and consumed.

Dosage: The appropriate dosage of guaco can vary depending on factors such as age, health status, and the specific preparation being used. It's important to follow the recommended dosage on the product label or consult with a qualified herbalist or healthcare professional for personalized guidance.

How to Use: Guaco tea is typically taken orally. It can be consumed on its own or mixed with honey or other herbal teas for added flavor.

Side Effects: Guaco is generally considered safe for most people when used in moderate amounts. However, some individuals may experience allergic reactions or digestive upset. It may also interact with certain medications or have adverse effects in individuals with certain health conditions. It's important to use guaco under the guidance of a healthcare professional and to discontinue use if any adverse effects occur.

Herban Iron:

Definition: Herban Iron is a dietary supplement designed to provide an easily absorbable form of iron to support healthy iron levels in the body. It's particularly beneficial for individuals with iron deficiency or anemia.

Ingredients: Herban Iron typically contains iron in the form of ferrous bisglycinate, which is a highly bioavailable and gentle form of iron that is less likely to cause digestive upset or constipation compared to other forms of iron. It may also contain other ingredients such as vitamin C to enhance iron absorption.

How to Prepare: Herban Iron is usually available in capsule or liquid form. Capsules are taken orally with water, while liquid forms may be mixed with water or juice before consumption. It's important to follow the recommended dosage on the product label.

Dosage: The appropriate dosage of Herban Iron depends on factors such as age, gender, and the severity of iron deficiency. It's important to consult with a healthcare professional to determine the correct dosage for individual needs.

How to Use: Herban Iron capsules are typically taken orally with water, while liquid forms may be mixed with water or juice before consumption. It's important to take Herban Iron as directed and to avoid taking it with dairy products, antacids, or other substances that may interfere with iron absorption.

Side Effects: While Herban Iron is generally considered safe for most people when used as directed, some individuals may experience mild side effects such as gastrointestinal discomfort or constipation. It's important to consult with a healthcare professional before starting any new supplement regimen, especially if you have underlying health conditions or are taking medications.

Cell Food:

Definition: Cell Food is a dietary supplement marketed as a highly oxygenating and alkalizing formula. It's claimed to support overall health and vitality by providing essential nutrients and oxygen to the cells.

Ingredients: The exact ingredients of Cell Food can vary depending on the brand, but it typically contains a proprietary blend of minerals, enzymes, electrolytes, and trace elements. Some common ingredients may include purified water, dissolved oxygen, seawater extract, and plant-based enzymes.

How to Prepare: Cell Food is usually available in liquid form and is typically taken orally. It can be consumed directly or diluted in water or juice before consumption.

Dosage: The dosage of Cell Food can vary depending on the specific product and individual needs. It's important to follow the recommended dosage on the product label or consult with a healthcare professional for personalized guidance.

How to Use: Cell Food is typically taken orally, either directly or mixed into water or juice. It's important to shake the bottle well before use and to store it according to the manufacturer's instructions.

Side Effects: Cell Food is generally considered safe for most people when used as directed. However, some individuals may experience mild digestive upset or allergic reactions to certain ingredients. It's essential to consult with a healthcare provider before starting any new supplement regimen, especially if you have underlying health conditions or are taking medications.

Chaparral:

Definition: Chaparral, scientifically known as Larrea tridentata, is a shrub native to the southwestern United States and northern Mexico. It has been used for centuries by Native American tribes for its medicinal properties and is commonly used in herbal medicine today.

Ingredients: Chaparral contains several bioactive compounds, including nordihydroguaiaretic acid (NDGA), flavonoids, lignans, and volatile oils. NDGA is believed to be the primary active compound responsible for many of chaparral's therapeutic effects.

How to Prepare: Chaparral can be prepared and consumed in various forms, including teas, tinctures, capsules, and topical preparations. To make tea, dried chaparral leaves are steeped in hot water for several minutes before being strained and consumed. Tinctures are prepared by steeping the herb in alcohol or vinegar to extract its active compounds.

Dosage: The appropriate dosage of chaparral can vary depending on the specific form and intended use. It's important to follow the recommended dosage on the product label or consult with a healthcare professional for personalized guidance.

How to Use: Chaparral tea or tincture is typically taken orally. It can also be applied topically to the skin for certain conditions. It's important to use chaparral products as directed and to discontinue use if any adverse effects occur.

Side Effects: Chaparral is generally considered safe for most people when used in moderate amounts. However, excessive intake or prolonged use may lead to liver toxicity or other adverse effects. It may also interact with certain medications or have adverse effects in individuals with certain health conditions. It's important to use chaparral under the guidance of a healthcare professional and to discontinue use if any adverse effects occur.

Hops:

Definition: Hops, scientifically known as Humulus lupulus, is a perennial climbing vine native to Europe, Asia, and North America. It is primarily known for its use in brewing beer but has also been used historically in traditional medicine for its potential health benefits.

Ingredients: Hops flowers contain various bioactive compounds, including bitter acids (such as humulone and lupulone), essential oils, flavonoids, and polyphenols. These compounds are believed to contribute to the herb's medicinal properties, including its potential as a sedative, relaxant, and digestive aid.

How to Prepare: Hops is typically consumed as an herbal tea, tincture, or in supplement form (such as capsules or tablets). To make tea, dried hops flowers are steeped in hot water for several minutes before being strained and consumed.

Dosage: The appropriate dosage of hops can vary depending on factors such as age, health status, and the specific preparation being used. It's important to follow the recommended dosage on the product label or consult with a qualified herbalist or healthcare professional for personalized guidance.

How to Use: Hops tea, tincture, or supplements are typically taken orally. It's often used to promote relaxation, relieve anxiety, and support sleep.

Side Effects: Hops is generally considered safe for most people when used in moderate amounts. However, some individuals may experience mild side effects such as drowsiness, gastrointestinal upset, or allergic reactions. It may also interact with certain medications or have adverse effects in individuals with certain health conditions, such as depression or hormone-sensitive conditions. It's important to use hops under the guidance of a healthcare professional and to discontinue use if any adverse effects occur.

Kelp:

Definition: Kelp refers to several species of large brown algae belonging to the Laminariales order. It is commonly found in underwater forests along rocky coastlines around the world. Kelp has been used for centuries in various cultures, particularly in East Asia, for its nutritional and medicinal properties.

Ingredients: Kelp is rich in various nutrients, including iodine, vitamins (such as vitamin K, vitamin C, and B vitamins), minerals (including calcium, magnesium, and potassium), antioxidants, and fiber. These nutrients are believed to contribute to the seaweed's potential health benefits, including its role in thyroid function, bone health, and immune support.

How to Prepare: Kelp is typically consumed dried, powdered, or in supplement form (such as capsules or tablets). It can also be used in cooking, particularly in soups, salads, and stir-fries. Kelp supplements are available in various forms, including powdered extracts, tablets, and liquid extracts.

Dosage: The appropriate dosage of kelp can vary depending on factors such as age, health status, and the specific preparation being used. It's important to follow the recommended dosage on the product label or consult with a qualified healthcare professional for personalized guidance.

How to Use: Kelp supplements are typically taken orally with water. They can be consumed as part of a daily nutritional regimen to support overall health and well-being. Kelp can also be incorporated into recipes as a flavorful and nutritious ingredient.

Side Effects: While kelp is generally considered safe for most people when consumed in moderate amounts, excessive intake of iodine-rich foods or supplements, including kelp, can lead to thyroid dysfunction or iodine toxicity. Some individuals may also be allergic to seaweed and experience allergic reactions. Pregnant or breastfeeding individuals should consult with a healthcare professional before using kelp supplements. It's important to use kelp under the guidance of a healthcare professional and to discontinue use if any adverse effects occur.

Cleavers:

Definition: Cleavers, scientifically known as Galium aparine, is a herbaceous annual plant native to Europe, North America, Asia, and Australia. It has a long history of use in traditional medicine for its potential health benefits.

Ingredients: Cleavers contains various bioactive compounds, including iridoid glycosides, flavonoids, tannins, and mucilage. These compounds are believed to contribute to the herb's medicinal properties, including its potential as a diuretic, lymphatic tonic, and mild astringent.

How to Prepare: Cleavers is typically consumed as an herbal tea, infusion, or in fresh salads. To make tea, dried cleavers leaves and stems are steeped in hot water for several minutes before being strained and consumed. It can also be used topically as a poultice or infused oil for skin conditions.

Dosage: The appropriate dosage of cleavers can vary depending on factors such as age, health status, and the specific preparation being used. It's important to follow the recommended dosage on the product label or consult with a qualified herbalist or healthcare professional for personalized guidance.

How to Use: Cleavers tea, infusion, or fresh leaves are typically taken orally. It's often used to support lymphatic drainage, promote urinary tract health, and soothe inflammation. Topically, cleavers can be applied to the skin to alleviate itching, irritation, or minor wounds.

Side Effects: Cleavers is generally considered safe for most people when consumed in moderate amounts. However, some individuals may experience allergic reactions or gastrointestinal upset. It may also interact with certain medications or have adverse effects in individuals with certain health conditions. Pregnant or breastfeeding individuals should consult with a healthcare professional before using cleavers supplements. It's important to use cleavers under the guidance of a healthcare professional and to discontinue use if any adverse effects occur.

Eucalyptus:

Definition: Eucalyptus refers to a genus of flowering trees and shrubs, primarily native to Australia but also found in other parts of the world. Eucalyptus essential oil, extracted from the leaves of certain species, has a long history of use in traditional medicine for its potential health benefits.

Ingredients: Eucalyptus essential oil contains various bioactive compounds, including eucalyptol (cineole), terpenes, and flavonoids. These compounds are believed to contribute to the oil's medicinal properties, including its potential as an expectorant, decongestant, antiseptic, and anti-inflammatory.

How to Prepare: Eucalyptus essential oil can be used in aromatherapy, diffused in the air, or diluted and applied topically to the skin. It can also be added to steam inhalations or chest rubs to help relieve respiratory symptoms.

Dosage: The appropriate dosage of eucalyptus essential oil can vary depending on factors such as age, health status, and the specific application being used. It's important to follow the recommended dosage on the product label or consult with a qualified aromatherapist or healthcare professional for personalized guidance.

How to Use: Eucalyptus essential oil can be used aromatically, topically, or internally, depending on the intended application. It's often used to alleviate respiratory congestion, soothe sore muscles, promote relaxation, and support overall well-being.

Side Effects: Eucalyptus essential oil is generally considered safe for most people when used appropriately. However, it can be toxic if ingested in large amounts and should not be applied directly to the skin without proper dilution. Some individuals may experience allergic reactions or respiratory irritation when exposed to eucalyptus oil. It's important to use eucalyptus oil with caution, especially around children and pets. Pregnant or breastfeeding individuals should consult with a healthcare professional before using eucalyptus oil. If any adverse effects occur, discontinue use and seek medical attention.

Feverfew:

Definition: Feverfew, scientifically known as Tanacetum parthenium, is a perennial herb native to Europe but also found in other parts of the world. It has a long history of use in traditional medicine, particularly in European folk medicine, for its potential health benefits.

Ingredients: Feverfew contains various bioactive compounds, including sesquiterpene lactones (such as parthenolide), flavonoids, and volatile oils. These compounds are believed to contribute to the herb's medicinal properties, including its potential as an anti-inflammatory, analgesic, and migraine prophylactic.

How to Prepare: Feverfew is typically consumed as an herbal tea, tincture, or in supplement form (such as capsules or tablets). To make tea, dried feverfew leaves and flowers are steeped in hot water for several minutes before being strained and consumed.

Dosage: The appropriate dosage of feverfew can vary depending on factors such as age, health status, and the specific preparation being used. It's important to follow the recommended dosage on the product label or consult with a qualified herbalist or healthcare professional for personalized guidance.

How to Use: Feverfew tea, tincture, or supplements are typically taken orally. It's often used to alleviate headaches, including migraines, and to support overall well-being.

Side Effects: Feverfew is generally considered safe for most people when used in moderate amounts. However, some individuals may experience mild side effects such as gastrointestinal upset or allergic reactions. It may also interact with certain medications or have adverse effects in individuals with certain health conditions, such as bleeding disorders or pregnancy. It's important to use feverfew under the guidance of a healthcare professional and to discontinue use if any adverse effects occur.

Ginseng:

Definition: Ginseng refers to several species of perennial plants belonging to the Panax genus, including Panax ginseng (Asian ginseng) and Panax quinquefolius (American ginseng). Ginseng has been used for centuries in traditional medicine, particularly in East Asia, for its potential health benefits.

Ingredients: Ginseng root contains various bioactive compounds, including ginsenosides, polysaccharides, and peptides. These compounds are believed to contribute to the herb's medicinal properties, including its potential as an adaptogen, immune enhancer, and cognitive booster.

How to Prepare: Ginseng is typically consumed as a powdered root, herbal tea, tincture, or in supplement form (such as capsules or tablets). To make tea, dried ginseng root slices are simmered in water for several minutes before being strained and consumed.

Dosage: The appropriate dosage of ginseng can vary depending on factors such as age, health status, and the specific preparation being used. It's important to follow the recommended dosage on the product label or consult with a qualified herbalist or healthcare professional for personalized guidance.

How to Use: Ginseng powder, tea, tincture, or supplements are typically taken orally. It's often used to support energy levels, enhance cognitive function, and promote overall well-being.

Side Effects: Ginseng is generally considered safe for most people when used in moderate amounts. However, some individuals may experience mild side effects such as insomnia, gastrointestinal upset, or headaches. It may also interact with certain medications or have adverse effects in individuals with certain health conditions, such as high blood pressure or diabetes. Pregnant or breastfeeding individuals should consult with a healthcare professional before using ginseng supplements. It's important to use ginseng under the guidance of a healthcare professional and to discontinue use if any adverse effects occur.

THE END